Essential Oils & Aromatherapy:

Balance Your Mind, Body, and Emotions

By John Gordon

John Gordon

The information in the following pages is broadly considered to be a truthful and accurate account of facts, and as such any inattention, use or misuse of the information in question by the reader will render any resulting actions solely under their purview. There are no scenarios in which the publisher or the original author of this work can be in any fashion deemed liable for any hardship or damages that may befall them after undertaking information described herein.

Additionally, the information in the following pages is intended only for informational purposes and should thus be thought of as universal. As befitting its nature, it is presented without assurance regarding its prolonged validity or interim quality. Trademarks that are mentioned are done without written consent and can in no way be considered an endorsement from the trademark holder.

Table of Contents

Introduction

Congratulations on purchasing your personal copy of *Essential Oils & Aromatherapy: Balance Your Mind, Body, and Emotions.* Thank you for doing so.

If you're interested in learning more about how you can keep both your mind and your body healthy far into your later years of life without the help of conventional medicine, you're not alone. It can sometimes feel like information is becoming increasingly less clear about what's healthy and what's unhealthy for our bodies. Conventional Western medicine is also known to be expensive, and people almost always prefer to avoid paying high medical costs if they can help it. In an attempt to keep your body pure and free of artificial substances, aromatherapy can be a great way to cure your ailments in a safe, cost-conscious, and effective way all at the same time.

This book is going to go over what aromatherapy is and how its use can greatly enhance your life. These enhancements can include ones that have to do with your mind's health, maintaining your body's ability to function, and even the ability to get a better night sleep on a regular basis. When all of your body can regulate itself consistently, the result is often an improved outlook on life as well as a more optimistic approach to life in general. The reality is that when you're bogged down by problems that negatively influence you in more ways than one, they can take a toll on your ability to focus on what truly matters in life. Aromatherapy can help to soothe your problems into oblivion, and will also create a calm and relaxing atmospheric backdrop for your life in the process.

While most of the chapters in this book are going to provide you with information about what aromatherapy is and its benefits, the last chapter of this book is going to discuss how you can begin to take the first steps towards integrating more aromatherapy techniques into your life. As with many other types of hobbies or disciplines, jumping into aromatherapy can at first seem a bit intimidating. What you're likely to find is that there are many different oils to choose from, and many methods to learn as well. How do you know what to choose? That's what the last chapter of this book will discuss. This way, you'll have a clear path that you can take towards using your aromatherapy knowledge and know-how.

There are plenty of books to choose from on the topic of aromatherapy. Thank you for choosing this one! Enjoy the rest of what this book, *Essential Oils & Aromatherapy: Balance Your Mind, Body, and Emotions* has to offer!

Chapter 1:
What is Aromatherapy?

If you're someone who already has a working knowledge of essential oils, then you may already know that aromatherapy involves the use of them. This chapter is going to focus on what aromatherapy is, and will also touch on when aromatherapy began. You're going to find that aromatherapy has a rich history, and its legitimacy as a type of medicine dates back to thousands of years ago. The ability of the practice of aromatherapy to survive to the present day is also an indicator of how powerful this practice can truly be.

Defining Aromatherapy

Also sometimes known as "essential oil therapy", aromatherapy can be best defined as both an art and a science. This may seem strange at first; however, the reason why it's defined in this manner is that the goal of aromatherapy is to promote health in mind, body, and even spirit. By strategically using essential oils in a particular way, aromatherapy can harmonize and balance any and all parts of the body that are out of sync with one another. Additionally, a key element of aromatherapy involves using essential oils to keep the body's healing processes healthy and intact. It's easy to conclude that when the body's immune system is functioning properly, a person's body will be able to fight and resist diseases with ease.

The Non-Invasive Nature of Aromatherapy

Unlike other types of medicinal treatments that claim to be completely free of harm for your body but still have risks associated with them, aromatherapy can be described as completely non-invasive and natural. Yes, some aromatherapy treatments do require that your internal body come into contact with an essential oil, but these types of treatments are typically going to be done by an aromatherapy professional who has a keen awareness of what he or she is doing. In other words, aromatherapy does not damage the liver or any other organs of the body, because it does not require the body to process anything except an aroma. This should be a relief to anyone who feels apprehensive about consuming prescription medication regularly.

How Essential Oils Aid in the Goals of Aromatherapy

This book is only going to discuss essential oils briefly, but it's important to understand that without essential oils, aromatherapy would not be possible. Essential oils are made up of chemicals that are natural to our environments. Through scientific use of these oils, aromatherapy can naturally influence the body. Most essential oils are ones that occur naturally, and they also are known to evaporate quickly once they're exposed to air. For this reason, aromatherapy will often involve the inhalation of these oils. If you think that different oils could have different effects on the body and the brain, you'd be correct. Aromatherapy also involves understanding how these oils interact with the body so that the correct oils can be used to achieve the desired results.

It's also important to note that different types of

essential oils are going to achieve a variety of outcomes for your mind, body, and spirit, depending on the oil that you choose to use during therapy. In other words, part of becoming a skilled aromatherapy practitioner involves knowing which oils do what. This book will help you to broaden your knowledge of the types of essential oils that you can use, and your experience dabbling with different types of essential oils will obviously help as well.

Aromatherapy and Your Emotions

In addition to being able to influence the brain and your body's daily functions, another impact that these oils can have is on your emotions. The primary way that our brains develop memories is through our sense of smell. Through the inhalation of essential oils during aromatherapy, it's possible to both bring positive memories to the surface, while also enabling your brain to clear out any unwanted memories that you may want to rid yourself of. For example, it is entirely possible that aromatherapy will bring an unpleasant emotion to the surface because your brain has already associated this smell with a certain memory. By being able to deal with memories that haunt your past, your brain will be able to more effectively process bad memories and get over them.

Due to the fact that essential oils can take a toll on your emotions, one of the first steps that you should take while practicing aromatherapy is to figure out which oils work for you and which do not. Experiment with certain oils to find out if any negatively influence your emotional demeanor. The goal of aromatherapy is to feel better, not worse. Additionally, if you do decide that you want to use aromatherapy to rid yourself of negative emotionally-charged memories of your past, the best advice is to do so with an aromatherapy professional by your side. This way, the professional will be able to guide you through your emotions in a safe way, and you won't run the risk of overwhelming yourself.

The Notion of Balance

It's also important to recognize that while aromatherapy is primarily touted as being able to target problems that are negatively influencing the body, it is also associated as being able to alleviate problems in the mind and the spirit as well. This positions aromatherapy as a comprehensive tool, rather than one that has one specific goal in mind. This makes sense, especially when you think about how a healthy body can often elevate your mental and spiritual capacities. The goal of aromatherapy is to feel fresh and rejuvenated after administering the techniques. If you do not feel this way after an aromatherapy session, it's safe to say that more practice is needed.

A Brief Background on Aromatherapy's History

Unlike other types of medicine that have been around for a long period of time, it's rather difficult to trace the origins of aromatherapy; however, there is a reason to believe that the Egyptians were the first ones to put essential oils to use. This is because the Egyptians were the first civilization to create oil distillation machines. These machines would extract the oils that are found in plants. The Egyptians are not the only civilization to be credited with popularizing aromatherapy. Both the ancient Chinese and Greek cultures also played a role in this development. The Chinese were the first people to infuse their oils, while the Greeks were known to use essential oils within their medical practices. The fact that three separate cultures developed facets of essential oil use suggests that many cultures in ancient times were very interested in how they could optimize the use of oils and get the most from their plants.

Chapter 2:
The Amazing Benefits of Aromatherapy

If the benefits of aromatherapy were not significant, then it's safe to say that this practice would have become obsolete centuries ago. Today, aromatherapy ranks among the oldest types of alternative medicinal techniques that exist in the world today. It's important that you understand what the benefits of aromatherapy are because understanding these techniques will likely motivate you to continue learning about how aromatherapy can enhance your quality of life. This chapter is going to discuss the immense benefits that aromatherapy can offer.

Aromatherapy Benefit 1: Anxiety Reduction

If you currently know very little about aromatherapy, one fact that you may have under your belt is that aromatherapy offers a great way for people to relieve stress. As anxiety continues to become a major reason for people's ailments all over the United States and even the world, it also becomes increasingly important for people to find new and innovative ways to reduce their stress. The secret behind why aromatherapy is an anxiety reducer has to do with the aroma that comes from the essential oils that are used throughout this process. These aromas can reduce stress so well that they've actually been termed "relaxants."

Aromatherapy Benefit 2: You'll Have More Energy

Another great benefit that aromatherapy can provide the body is that it's known to give the body greater levels of energy. These days, people are constantly on the move. Everyone seems to have different vices that they use in the hopes of keeping their energy high and alert throughout the day, but often these sources can be detrimental to the body over the long-term. Some of these vices include drinking coffee, smoking, and even consuming sugary energy drinks. Aromatherapy can offer a unique and refreshing take on how to keep the body energetic and active, because aromatherapy does not require the body to actually consume calories, carbohydrates, or fat. Of course, using essential oils that are appropriate for relaxing may not be the best ones to use when your goal is to have energy and wake up. When you're using aromatherapy as a way to become more energized, the best ones to use are pepper, rosemary, sage, or cardamom.

Aromatherapy Benefit 3: You'll Heal More Quickly

Every day, our bodies are bombarded by bacteria, some of which can cause the body to become sick if we're not prepared to fight them. There are two primary reasons why our bodies can fail at protecting itself against harmful bacteria. The first one is poor diet and health. This is an aspect of your health over which you have control. If you do not put healthy food and energy into your body, there's less of a chance that your body is going to be able to function as efficiently as possible. Some great essential oils that can be helpful during the healing process include rosehip, lavender, and calendula.

The other primary factor that can influence your body's ability to heal and protect itself is age. As we get older, our bodies' immune systems naturally begin to slow down the longer we're alive. This is inevitable, and in contrast to maintaining a healthy diet, we do not have control over the body's deterioration through time; however, aromatherapy has been known to help the body during the healing process, even for older folks. Aromatherapy can speed up the body's healing process because it encourages greater levels of oxygen to flow throughout the body. Additionally, certain essential oils have anti-microbial properties within them. You can think of these properties as being similar to a soap that you'd use to wash your hands. When you use these types of essential oils, you're able to protect the area of your body that is in the process of healing. In fact, it's not uncommon for people who practice aromatherapy to participate in aromatherapy sessions during post-surgery or while recovering from an accident. This speaks to the power of aromatherapy.

Aromatherapy Benefit 4: Helps to Kick those

Headaches

Headaches often go hand-in-hand with experiencing high levels of stress, so it makes sense that aromatherapy can help to reduce these as well. Additionally, there are plenty of ways that you can reduce headaches via artificial medicine; however, aromatherapy can offer a fabulous alternative to ending your headaches with natural medicine. Sometimes, people also look to neck and head massages as a way to alleviate headaches; however, these types of massages often come with an expensive price tag. Aromatherapy offers a relatively inexpensive way to alleviate even the most intense headaches and has also been known to prevent the development of headaches in the future. A few common essential oils that are known to combat headaches and migraines efficiently include eucalyptus, ginger, and sandalwood.

Aromatherapy Benefit 5: Sleep Maintenance

Another fabulous benefit of aromatherapy is that it aids

in the regulation of sleep. There are countless reasons why people have trouble sleeping, ones that have to do with stress, and ones that have to do with other underlying problems. If you've ever experienced a sleepless night yourself, then you're already aware of how a lack of sleep can make you feel the next day. People who do not get enough sleep at night due to restlessness typically feel lethargic, unproductive, and irritable on a day-to-day basis. Even though the pharmaceutical companies may claim that their medicines have no side effects, sleeping aids, in general, are known to be incredibly addictive. Aromatherapy is a great alternative for anyone who suffers from the inability to sleep, without the dangers that prescription medicine often present.

There are plenty of other benefits that aromatherapy can provide, but the ones that were just presented in this chapter are often considered to be the most important ones. When your body can relax and rejuvenate itself properly, the result is a better quality of life and greater enjoyment on a daily basis. What's truly amazing is that even though these benefits are readily available to anyone who seeks them out, a number of people who use aromatherapy techniques is quite small. These benefits are proven, which is why you should be looking to implement aromatherapy techniques into your daily life as soon as possible.

Chapter 3:
The Best Essential Oils to Use During Aromatherapy

As you have already seen after reading the previous chapter, there are many different essential oils that you can use within the art of aromatherapy. Often, the type of essential oil that you use during an aromatherapy session is going to depend on the purpose that you have. This chapter is going to dive more deeply into the types of essential oils that you should be using, depending on what you're looking to accomplish. After reading this chapter, you should be able to use it as a guide whenever you're looking to use aromatherapy for a specific purpose. Even people who have been practicing aromatherapy for a while can agree that being able to memorize which essential oils should be used for what takes time. This chapter will also briefly discuss the cost of aromatherapy, and how this cost differs from other types of medicinal practices that are out there.

The Most Popular Aromatherapy Essential Oils

When you're first starting out learning about aromatherapy, it's best to begin by learning about the most common types of essential oils that practitioners of aromatherapy typically use. There are always going to be obscure varieties of oil with which you can experiment, but without an awareness of the basic types, you'll never begin to advance. Let's take a look at some of the most popular essential oils and their uses.

Tea Tree Oil

Many people who swear by the benefits of aromatherapy often claim that tea tree oil is the most important essential oil that exists. It's often stated that if you only own one essential oil for aromatherapy, tea tree oil should be what's in your possession. Tea tree oil is known for being able to aid in the body's healing processes by bolstering the immune system. It's also known to combat infections well. When you're using tea tree oil during aromatherapy, feel free to either inhale the oil or blend it directly into the skin. In addition to fighting infections, tea tree oil can also alleviate pain that comes with a burn to the skin. It also can help to cure dandruff (when combined with shampoo) and Athlete's foot.

Lavender Oil

Similar to tea tree oil, lavender is an essential oil that's often used in aromatherapy. It's mainly used to help in relaxation, but it has some other uses as well. For example, using lavender oil can help the body to fight colds, severe headaches, and even the flu. Some people use lavender oil as a replacement for deodorant, believe it or not. There are multiple ways that you can apply lavender oil to the body, but one of the more relaxing techniques involves adding lavender oil to a bath. Lavender's relaxing aroma is sure to enhance a bath and relax the body. Lastly, some people also spritz lavender oil on their pillow prior to falling asleep at night. This often has the result of bringing individuals a better night's sleep. It's important to note that some people are allergic to lavender oil. If you've never used lavender oil before and you notice your skin developing a rash once you start to use it, discontinue using it.

Lemon Oil

The last popular oil that we're going to discuss is lemon oil. Often, the first quality that people will notice about lemon oil is its refreshing and clean scent. While this is reason enough to start using lemon oil for aromatherapy purposes, some other attractive qualities of lemon oil include aiding the mind in concentration, helping the body digest more smoothly, and it also aids in the reduction of arthritis and bad skin. Another great quality of lemon oil is that it can help reduce cellulite for people who have it. The crisp and refreshing scent of the oil is also known to improve mood.

Now that we've gone over three of the most popular essential oils, we're now going to go over which oils are best for some common ailments that are frequently cured using aromatherapy techniques. This way, you will be able to reference these oils and use them when these ailments arise in your own life.

The Best Essential Oils for Anxiety

As we've already noted, anxiety is one of the leading problems that face Americans and other people all over the world today. When you're looking to treat your anxiety with aromatherapy, you should consider doing so with the following oils:

1. Chamomile: Chamomile can be found in many products that people use on a daily basis. Many people describe chamomile as having a floral yet fruity scent to it, along with subtle notes of apple in it.

2. Lavender: Lavender is another oil that is great for curing anxiety, even anxiety that can be described as intense, including panic attacks.

3. Rose: Rose oil is going to be able to provide the body with similar effects that lavender oil can; however, rose oil is also going to provide emotional stability as well. In particular, rose oil can be used during aromatherapy to fight anxiety and the depression that can come with it.

The Best Essential Oils for Digestion

There's a chance that you've never considered the fact that essential oils can be used to promote digestive health. This is a lesser-known benefit that essential oils can have on the body during aromatherapy. Additionally, it's important to note that for these digestive oils, you can consume a drop or two orally. Some of the best essential oils for digestion include the following:

1. Ginger: When the body is constipated, ginger oil aids in relieving the body of this pressure and discomfort by invigorating the digestive tract.

2. Cardamom: Did you know that cardamom is considered to be part of the ginger plant family? Similar to ginger, the flavor and scent of cardamom are slightly sweeter and comforting than the powerful properties of ginger.

3. Fennel: Fennel oil can be used to combat feelings of

nausea or gassy intestines. If you've ever eaten fennel, then you're already aware of the earthy and root-like flavor that it has. The oil is quite similar to this flavor.

The Cost of Essential Oils

Now that we've gone over two major ways that you can use specific essential oils, let's turn our attention to something that is bound to cross your mind at some point. Yes, it is the subject of cost. Of course, it's safe to say that everyone who dabbles in aromatherapy would love nothing more than to have every variety of essential oil at their disposal, but the reality is that the cost of having a diverse array of essential oils to personally choose from can become rather expensive.

On average, a fifteen-ounce bottle of essential oil will cost you between twenty and twenty-five dollars. Of course, some varieties of oil are more expensive than others, depending on what you choose to purchase and how difficult it is to extract this oil from its source. Due to the fact that these oils are often far from cheap, it's best to do some research prior to purchasing. If there's no logical reason why an essential oil is priced higher than you expect, then it's best to proceed with skepticism.

Chapter 4:
Understanding How Aromatherapy Can Help You

In addition to the benefits that we've already gone over in chapter two, there are plenty of other benefits that aromatherapy can provide you that go beyond basic knowledge and understanding. This chapter is going to seek to broaden your understanding of how aromatherapy can help you remedy problems that are a bit more obscure than the basic benefits that aromatherapy can provide. After reading this chapter, the hope is that your foundation of knowledge regarding how essential oils can help you will be broadened and much more comprehensive.

Regulating Arthritis and Inflammation with Aromatherapy

Arthritis is a form of inflammation, that often cripples older people. While some forms of arthritis can be rather benign, other forms are known to cause the body extreme pain in the joints where the arthritis is occurring. Most doctors will administer drugs that can ease the pain that comes along with the development of arthritis, but aromatherapy is a scientifically-proven technique that you can use to fight arthritis as well. The specific oils that can be used during aromatherapy to alleviate all types of inflammation include frankincense, wintergreen, and orange. You may not currently think about how inflamed your body's joints are. Using essential oils as a way to reduce inflammation may start to help you realize where any joint pain is occurring.

Memory Loss that Comes with Age

Another affliction that can take an older person by storm is the inability to remember important life events and things. Even though it's been proven that ailments such as Alzheimer's can be avoided by eating certain foods, the beginning signs of Alzheimer's can often creep up on a person before they even realizing what's happening. Instead of succumbing to an ailment that is sure to cause you emotional pain, a better option would be to prevent this problem through the use of essential oils. Some studies have even shown that younger children who have aromatherapy administered on them can retain larger amounts of information immediately after treatment. Some of the best essential oils that can combat dementia include sage oil, Cyprus oil, and basil oil.

Healing Scrapes and Cuts

Do you know what's in topical treatment medicines like Neosporin? Neither do I. Another great way to use essential oils and aromatherapy is as topical medicine that can aid in the healing of scrapes and cuts. This is an especially good use of essential oils for children. There are countless essential oils that contain antibacterial and anti-swelling properties, which is why they can be the perfect remedy for small to medium-sized abrasions. Additionally, essential oils are known to be able to penetrate the skin and heal any blood vessels that may have become injured as well. Lastly, it's important to note that you can use essential oils to heal scars that have formed on the skin. The best oils for scrapes, cuts, and even scars include myrrh oil, cedarwood oil, or almond oil.

Essential Oils for Menstruation

Instead of going to the store and purchasing a synthetic product to help with menstrual cramps, why not seek out essential oils next time? While women can develop cramps for a variety of reasons before and during their menstruation cycle, a large majority of these cramps are caused by a compression or tightness in the lower stomach region. For this reason, you can opt to rub some essential oil on the lower stomach area. You'll likely find that this will reduce your cramps and calm the body a bit. Conversely, you can also place a cloth of some type on the back of the neck, and add some essential oils to that as well. Some of the best oils for soothing PMS and menstrual-related problems include cypress oil, sage oil, and peppermint oil.

Aromatherapy Can Ease General Body Pain

If you're young and reading this book, then you may not believe that people actually begin to experience general body pain on a daily basis when they start to age, but it's true.

After a long day at work or being outside on the weekend with your kids, it's not uncommon for middle-aged and older-aged people to feel a dull pain in their knees, back, or shoulders. The muscles and joints that are associated with these areas of the body need some love and kindness after strenuous activity. This is where aromatherapy can become beneficial. Oils such as clove, citrus, and jojoba can quicken blood circulation, bringing relief to these areas of the body that are feeling strained and overworked.

Using Aromatherapy to Cure Congestion

The last way that you can use aromatherapy to cure common maladies is when you're feeling congested. If you live in an area of the world that experiences the changing of seasons, then it's likely that you've felt the sneezes and coughs coming on that frequently accompany the falling of the leaves or the dying of flowers. When you're looking to use aromatherapy techniques to rid yourself of a cold or congestion, the best way to do this is by taking a bath and then adding the oils to the bath. Some of the best oils to use when you're feeling congested include eucalyptus or sesame seed. If you do decide to take a bath using these oils, it's important that you do not accidentally splash yourself in the eye. Eucalyptus oil, in particular, is known to be an eye irritant.

After reading this chapter, you should now have an even broader understanding of how essential oils and aromatherapy can help to keep your body functioning at its highest level, without the use of artificial medicines or treatments. As you can see, aromatherapy can cure a long list of ailments that go far beyond simply being used as a way to complement relaxation. More importantly, if you currently do not use a lot of medicine, but instead choose to not do anything when you experience the ailments that were presented in this chapter, then it's obvious that aromatherapy could greatly enhance your life. Using aromatherapy on a frequent basis is sure to increase your quality of life. This will allow to feel more sure of yourself and secure on a daily basis because you'll know that you're taking care of your own wellness first and foremost.

Chapter 5:
Aromatherapy Techniques from Beginner to Advanced

At this point in the book, it's clear that you have plenty of knowledge regarding the best essential oils to use when you're attempting to achieve a concrete goal; however, we have yet to discuss how to actually implement aromatherapy when you're ready to start using the oils that you've purchased. That's what this chapter will cover. After reading this chapter, you will have a wide range of techniques at your disposal that will allow you start feeling like you can perform aromatherapy yourself. In other words, these techniques will range from beginner ones to more advanced ones. Even if you're not completely confident that you'd be able to implement all of the techniques that this chapter lays out, you'll at least know how aromatherapy techniques work.

Aromatherapy Technique 1: Body Massage

If you were to seek professional aromatherapy, you'd probably start by seeking out a professional who applies the essential oils to the body through massage techniques. The amount of oil that an aromatherapy specialist will use on the body during a massage will likely depend on your age. For example, if an aromatherapy specialist were performing a massage on a child or young adult, he or she would probably use between three to six drops of essential oils. On the other hand, if the aromatherapy specialist was massaging an adult, they could use as little as fifteen drops of oil to sixty drops of oil. If you're unsure of how much oil your aromatherapist is using, it's best to ask. Additionally, if you have a preference as to the amount of essential oil you'd like to receive during your massage, you should also bring this up with the specialist as well. It's very unlikely that the therapist will use only essential oil while performing the massage. Instead, he or she will likely use a blend of essential oils and another herbal or vegetable oil.

Aromatherapy Technique 2: A Bath

Similar to an aromatherapy massage, an aromatherapy bath may also be a type of aromatherapy technique with which you're already familiar. You can easily perform an aromatherapy bath yourself, but there are also places that exist that will create an aromatherapy bath experience for you. Either way that you bath is prepared, there should be between two to twelve drops of essential oils in the water. Unlike the massage oil method, it's important that the essential oil is mixed with something else before you get into it. You have the option of mixing the essential oil with things like bath gel or polysorbate. Even though you may not have heard of polysorbate before, it's simply a thickening agent that is used in many cosmetic products.

Combining the oil with a thickening agent will help to bring out the truest essence of the essential oil that you're using. Of course, if you decide to make an aromatherapy bath at home, do not forget to light your candles and purchase a bath pillow so that you can achieve a truly relaxing experience. If you do not have gel or polysorbate, do not fret. Vegetable oil is an easily accessible alternative.

Aromatherapy Technique 3: Facial and Body

Cream

An aromatherapy cream can be bought in most natural retail stores, or you can always try your hand at making it yourself. Without careful knowledge of how to make aromatherapy cream, it's best to purchase products that you know have the proper amounts of oil and other ingredients in it. For example, if you're looking for an essential oil face cream, but know that your skin is more sensitive in nature, then it would be best to find yourself a cream that only has between a half drop and 1 full drop of essential oil in it. If you add more than this, you'll run the risk of burning yourself. In fact, even if you're someone who does not have overly sensitive skin, you would only want to use an essential oil face cream with around one to two and a half drops of oil in it. These creams, whether they're for your face or for the rest of your body, can have an incredibly soothing effect on the skin.

Aromatherapy Technique 4: The Diffusion Process

Diffusion means to simply spread something around, so when it comes to aromatherapy, diffusion means to spread the scent of an essential oil throughout a space as a way to optimize its aroma. To do this, you need to purchase something known as a diffuser. A diffuser is going to spread an essential oil's aroma throughout a room or space and will save you from having to diffuse the oil manually. Even though the term "diffuser" sounds fancy, they are pretty simple to use. To use a diffuser, follow these steps:

1. Remove the tub of the diffuser from the diffuser itself

2. Fill the tub of the diffuser with lukewarm water

2. Mix in between ten to fifteen drops of your preferred essential oil

3. Place the tub back on the diffuser, making sure that it snugly fits into place

4. Click the "power" button on your diffuser. The location of this button will depend on the model that you choose to purchase

That's all there is to getting started with using a diffuser. As with any product that can be considered a luxury rather than a necessity, you'll be able to find diffusers that cost upwards of one hundred dollars if you were to look for them; however, a more reasonable estimate for the price of a diffuser is probably between thirty to fifty dollars.

This chapter has provided you with countless ways to start thinking about how you can easily integrate aromatherapy into your own life. Remember, if you do not yet feel comfortable experimenting with aromatherapy techniques on your own, you should at the very least seek out an aromatherapist who can guide you and make you feel more comfortable with the aromatherapy process. On average, a one-hour session with an aromatherapist can cost around fifty dollars. Sure, you may not want to pay this much money for aromatherapy treatments consistently, but going to an aromatherapist at least one time will allow you to become more comfortable with what aromatherapy has to offer.

Chapter 6:
Tips on How to Practice Aromatherapy at Home

Now that you have a more comprehensive understanding of aromatherapy techniques and how you can use essential oils effectively, this next chapter is going to go over how you can start to use aromatherapy in your own home. These techniques are slightly different from the techniques that were presented in the previous chapter, but they are still going to be able to achieve similar results. The only difference here is that you'll be able to implement these techniques yourself. You won't need to rely on anyone except yourself as you move towards performing aromatherapy in your home.

Direct Inhalation of Essential Oils

The first at-home way that we're going to discuss in regard to aromatherapy consists of essential oil inhalation. This is an extremely simple technique. You have a few options when you want to inhale an essential oil directly. These options include:

1. **Direct Inhalation from the Bottle:** Rather than directly inhaling the essential oil from the bottle that you purchased or made yourself, it's best to first create a solution of at least three different essential oils. Begin by pouring this tri-blend of oils into your own bottle. Once you've done that, use your hand to waft the scent from the bottle towards your nose. You can repeat this technique for as many as four times per day if you wish.

2. **Direct Inhalation from Bottle with Salt:** Another variation of the previous technique involves mixing your three oils with salts, and then wafting this solution towards your nose. Similar to the previous technique, you can perform this technique up to four times per day.

3. **Direct Inhalation from Your Palm:** To perform this technique, place between six to eight drops of one essential oil type onto one of your hands. Rub your hands together, and then you can sniff the oil directly from your

palms. Not only will your nose thank you for using this technique, but your hands will too.

4. Direct Inhalation from A Cloth or Cotton Ball: When using a cloth, you can smell the essential oil or blend of essential oils from the cloth itself; however, if you choose to dab the essential oil onto a cotton ball, it's best to use a wafting technique. An aroma that's placed on the cotton ball will be much stronger than an aroma that's placed on a cloth.

5. Direct Inhalation from an Inhaler Tube: When you're on the go or traveling, but still want to be able to relax by using essential oils, an inhaler tube is a fabulous option. This tube is specifically designed for people who are on-the-go. These tubes are roughly the size of a larger Chapstick. They're made of plastic and contain a small section of cotton that fits inside of the tube. To use, pour your essential oil onto the cotton ball, and then re-attach the plastic lid that also comes with the tube. When you're ready to use the tube, you can simply take off the cap, pinch one of your nostrils, and bring the tube towards the unplugged nostril. Sniff as needed.

I wasn't joking when I said that you have plenty of options when it comes to how you want to inhale your essential oil. When you're deciding on which technique you should use, the best advice is to try all of them before choosing. You may find that one technique is too strong for your liking, or that another one does not emit a strong enough aroma for your personal taste. You can also adapt these techniques in any way that you like, to achieve results that are perfect for you.

Using a Spritzer in Your Home

In addition to directly inhaling an essential oil, many people also opt to use the technique of spritzing while they're in the confines of their own home. The only tool that you're going to need when you want to spritz is a spray bottle; however, you're not going to be spritzing essential oils alone into it. Instead, you're going to be adding both water and essential oils to the bottle. You can also add a substance that will thicken this mixture to the bottle with the water and the oil. Proponents of this technique will typically spritz refreshing oils into rooms of their home to make them smell refreshing before company comes over. Others have also been known to spritz lavender oil on their pillow before going to sleep at night, as this will create a soothing aroma before bed.

While you can of course experiment with the different types of oils that you want to use in the spritz bottle, consider using between ten to fifteen drops of essential oil per single ounce of water. Additionally, be sure to shake the bottle prior to spritzing it anywhere, so that everything blends nicely. In addition to freshening a room and being good for pre-sleep use, aromatherapy spritzers can also be used as an alternative to body spray or to make it easier to breathe in your home. While a spritzer cannot be exactly compared to the functionality of an electric diffuser, a spray bottle can also take the place of an electric one if you're light on cash or are not ready to purchase a diffuser outright.

Aromatherapy Via Steam Inhalation

The last technique that this chapter is going to cover that you can perform at home on yourself is steam inhalation. To do this, you would first boil water on the stove. Once the water is boiling, mix in between four to seven drops of essential oil. Next, remove this mixture from the stove. Place the water solvent into a plastic or glass bowl, before bringing the bowl to a place where your head can hover above it. Drape a towel over your head, and allow the steam from the bowl of water to lift the aromas of the essential oils towards your face. Make sure to keep your eyes closed while performing this technique. Draping the towel over your head will keep the steam concentrated around your face, allowing the essential oil to coat the towel like a dew. When you're suffering from congestion, this technique can be a perfect remedy for those clogged lungs or throat. Steam inhalation is also sometimes used to cure sinus infections as well.

Chapter 7:
How Essential Oils Can Improve Your Mental Health

In addition to being able to cure ailments within the body, aromatherapy is also known to be a great way to cure problems within the mind. So far, this book has mainly discussed the physical benefits that have been scientifically proven to exist through aromatherapy techniques. We have yet to discuss how the smell of certain fragrances can alter the mind. This chapter is going to cover how aromatherapy can successfully change our states of consciousness for the better.

The Depression Epidemic

In the United States, it's been reported that at least 10 million adults have expressed feeling depressed to some degree within the past year. This number is nothing to scoff at; however, it can sometimes seem as if too many people look to prescription medicine in the hope of extinguishing depression from their minds. The truth of the matter is that many people suffer from depression because of the circumstances in their life. Instead of changing those circumstances, many people opt to take the "easier" route of ingesting prescription medication. While not all medication is ineffective, practices like aromatherapy can do wonders for a person who does not truly need a prescription medication in their life. Imagine how much less money the pharmaceutical companies had if people took more time to learn about aromatherapy and how it can make an impact on the mind for the better.

Our Emotions and Our Immune System

Many people may not think that our mental facilities are impacted by the healthiness of our physical body; however, there is strong evidence suggesting the contrary. In fact, it's now been proven that negative emotions such as anger or depression are linked to a less effective immune system. Without getting too technical, what this essentially means is that the health of our immune system can and does influence our mind's sense of happiness throughout our daily lives.

With this being the case, it makes logical sense that

we'd want to try and make our immune systems as strong as possible, if only because our mind will feel as healthy as our immune system does. This is how essential oils can help. Known to strengthen the immune system, essential oils that aid in the preservation of our immune system are also targeting our emotions and mind's health at the same time. This should incentivize anyone who is thinking about using more aromatherapy techniques to do so. Not only will using essential oils have a positive impact on the body; they will undoubtedly have a positive impact on the mind as well.

Aromatherapy and Depression

Depression can be a side effect of anxiety, or it can be a problem in and of itself. Even though aromatherapy can certainly aid in the maintenance of depression, it's important to note that you should not attempt to treat depression through the techniques of aromatherapy alone. Instead, you should create a long-term health plan that will use aromatherapy within it. Admittedly, plenty of more research needs to be done when it comes to figuring out exactly why aromatherapy can help to treat depression; however, plenty of people can attest to the fact that aromatherapy does, in fact, work to fight against depression and feelings of immense sadness.

The Best Essential Oil for Treating Depression

As we've already seen, not all essential oils are created equal. Some of the best essential oils to use when you're looking to defeat depression include the following:

1. Bergamot Oil: In 2011, a study in Thailand was conducted on rats. The result of this study found that the aroma from bergamot essential oil effectively decreased stress that the rats were feeling. Even though people are not quite sure why bergamot oil is known to treat depression, its citrusy and floral qualities are known to awaken the spirit and stimulate the mind into a state of greater contentment.

2. Ylang-Ylang Oil: Ylang-Ylang oil has more of a banana-like aroma to it than does bergamot oil. The name of this oil might be enough to stave off depression in someone and instead give them a nice laugh, but this oil is no joke when it comes to being able to calm the mind and ease the senses. One reason why ylang-ylang oil can help someone who is suffering from depression is that this oil has a sedative quality to it. In fact, some studies have shown that ylang-ylang oil can fight off emotions that go beyond depression. These include jealousy, anger, and even mental problems that have to do with low self-worth.

How to Use Aromatherapy for Depression

The ways in which you can use aromatherapy to treat depression are similar to the methods that we've already discussed in previous chapters; however, you can still get creative when you're using aromatherapy as a way to treat depression in rather innovative ways. For example, you can try to curb your depression while you sleep. To do this, simply set up your diffuser and place some anti-depressing essential oils into the diffuser before you fall asleep at night. There's no risk in allowing your diffuser to work throughout the night. Another great method involves placing anti-depressant essential oils in strategic places of the body. Some of these places include the bottoms of the feet, the stomach, and the backs of the neck or ears.

You do not have to live with your depression. This book is not advocating that aromatherapy will be able to completely cure the depression that you're facing, but aromatherapy can certainly help you in your pursuits to end your depressive state. Even if you're not depressed, we all get down in the dumps every once in a while. Having these techniques at your disposal can be the difference between a night of sulking and a night of feeling sad, but knowing that the sad feelings will come and go. Again, do not feel like you need to treat your depression on your own. Aromatherapy can be a great supplement to other types of treatment you might be receiving.

Chapter 8:
Aromatherapy and Ayurveda

Perhaps you've heard the term Ayurveda before in the past, but there's also a chance that you have not. The term is becoming more popular in modern day society, perhaps because of the prevalence of yoga and the surge in interest regarding self-healing methods. This chapter is going to discuss exactly what Ayurveda is, and will also get into how Ayurveda is associated with aromatherapy.

What is Ayurveda?

Ayurveda can best be described as a type of holistic medicine. More importantly, it's technically the world's oldest medicine in the course of history. "Holistic" in this case refers to the fact that this type of medicine can cure the entire body. In other words, it's not medicine that is used to target one specific problem or area but can instead heal all aspects of a person's body, including their mind and spirit. The logic behind Ayurveda is that everything in the body is connected in some way to one another. The goal of Ayurveda is to treat entire systems of the body while keeping in mind that truly everything in this world has a relationship with any and all other living beings.

In addition to seeing the entire body as a cohesive unit, Ayurvedic medicine also works under the assumption that every living thing in the entire world is connected to one another in some manner. While Ayurveda began in India roughly three-thousand years ago, today it is formally considered to be what's known as CAM, or complementary and alternative form of medicine in the United States. Within Ayurveda, it's even believed that living things that have already died and perished are connected to the current order of things that are living and breathing. When your energy, including your body's physical health and wellness, is out of sync with the rest of the universe, the idea is that you're going to become physically sick. As you may have guessed, Ayurveda also contains elements that promote living a healthy lifestyle from a spiritual perspective as well.

John Gordon

So...How Does Aromatherapy Fit into the Mix?

The practice of Ayurveda has been implementing the use of aromatherapy from its onset. When Ayurveda was first developed, people would typically burn wood as a way to benefit from the aroma that was being emanated from it. The Indian people and the Egyptian people were the first societies that began to use aromatherapy in this small and rather insignificant manner, but other cultures soon followed their lead. Most notably, it was the ancient Greeks who expanded the use of aromatherapy from the practice of burning wood to include the burning of olive oil to achieve the same goals. Over this time period, you can say that the burning of essential oils was being perfected and experimented with. Even in ancient Chinese culture, history sees a reliance on essential oils as a healing practice very early on.

Even though Ayurvedic medicine does go beyond the scope of simply smelling essential oils in the hope that this will lead to full body health, it's important to note that within Ayurvedic medicine there are countless ways to achieve medicinal healing through the powers that the essence of aromatic oils can bring. Ayurveda's relationship with aromatherapy brings up an excellent point regarding aromatherapy in general. At the core of aromatherapy treatment lies the fact that most if not all of these oils are being derived from something that is completely natural. This is perhaps the strongest link between aromatherapy and Ayurveda.

How Does Ayurveda Implement Aromatherapy Techniques?

Even though a deep discussion of Ayurveda treatments is largely beyond the scope of this book, if you've ever felt skeptical about the usefulness of modern medicine and more importantly the vast side effects that typically accompany modern medicine, then perhaps you should look into expanding Ayurveda techniques into your own life. Additionally, you could also look to use aromatherapy as a way to expand your knowledge of Ayurveda as well, simply by understanding how Ayurveda implements the techniques of aromatherapy. Ayurveda uses aromatherapy in some of the following ways:

1. **Natural Teas, Powders, and Pills:** It's not uncommon to see Ayurveda treatments in stores that advocate for the consumption of natural teas, powders and pills. Often, when you look at the ingredients of these concoctions, you'll find that some type of natural oil has been used to fulfill its creation. Many of these oils have effects that are calming, or that can serve as anti-inflammatory agents. Others are used to decongest the body's nasal passages and systems, and still, more are used to boost the body's immune system as a way to fight any bacteria that might try to infiltrate the body during the colder months of the year.

2. **Steam Treatment:** Another primary facet of Ayurveda treatment involves steam therapy. The difference between these methods and the method that we discussed in the chapter regarding aromatherapy techniques is that Ayurveda treatments will typically involve an entire bath of steam. If you recall, this differs from the aromatherapy

technique that we discussed, which primarily focuses on channeling steam towards the face. Additionally, while aromatherapy does not actively use whole plants in its application, Ayurveda does. Some steam treatments involve bringing entire plants into the bath so that the patient can inhale the aroma from these plants; however, essential oils are also used.

3. Nasya: Nasya is a medicinal treatment that involves the injection of essential oil blends directly into the nose. This is considered to be an aromatherapy technique; however, this book does not advise you to perform nasya on your own. Any time that aromatherapy involves consuming an essential oil into the body, you should seek out professional help. The effects of essential oils within the body can result in nausea or sickness, when not administered properly.

4. Incense Therapy: Ayurveda techniques include incense therapy, which can be described as a method that's meant to be a remedy for protecting the immune system and for purification as well. While incense is obviously different from the way in which aromatherapy is used, both incense therapy and aromatherapy are often used with to achieve the common goal of purification and sanitation as well. Incense therapy is also used for relieving anxiety and emotional stress that can sometimes weigh on the mind. The general mode of thought is that while even though incense therapy is not quite the same as aromatherapy, they have similarities within this realm.

As you can see, aromatherapy and Ayurveda have a relationship with one another that dates back thousands of years. Even though Ayurveda medicinal techniques do sometimes use plants and herbs rather than exclusively essential oils, the techniques of Ayurveda and aromatherapy do collide every now and again. The scope of this book is not meant to focus much on Ayurveda medicine; however, if you have a natural inclination towards natural medicine and ways to keep yourself healthy without risking damage to your liver through the consumption of prescription medication, then learning more about Ayurveda is surely going to be of interest to you.

Chapter 9:
Mistakes to Avoid While Initiating Yourself

As with any other hobby or specialty, there is a right way to do things and a wrong way to do things when it comes to aromatherapy. This chapter is going to go over what you shouldn't do when using essential oils for an intended purpose. The hope is that after reading this chapter, you will have the wherewithal to avoid these same mistakes yourself. More importantly, when it comes to aromatherapy, it's important to keep in mind that you're going to have oil administered to your body. If you're not aware of some mistakes that people have made in the past, you could end up injuring yourself. No one wants that to happen.

Aromatherapy Mistake 1: Not Checking the Label

A key beginner mistake that people make when they're just beginning to use essential oils involves not checking the label on the packaging prior to purchasing a bottle of essential oils. Many essential oils that exist are not entirely pure. Some are made up of artificial chemicals that can hurt the skin, while others are made with cheaply grown materials that you would be better off without. Just like when you go to an organic food store, the best essential oils are the pure ones. If that means that you have to pay a few more dollars for the purer version of the oil, so be it.

Aromatherapy Mistake 2: Mixing Oil with Water

Many people think that adding copious amounts of water to oil will help to make the oil less irritable for more sensitive parts of the body, but this is not the case. Oil and water do not naturally mix. This is why it's important to mix your oils with other oil, such as vegetable or almond oil. As we've already discussed, you can also always mix the oil with something that will serve as a thickening agent to the essential oil as well. Rest assured that it's unlikely that you'll do significant damage to the body if you do end up mixing an essential oil with only water; however, there are plenty of stories out there involving irritation caused by mixing water with oil. For example, if you decide to give a child an aromatherapy bath, their skin is likely going to be more sensitive to the oil than perhaps yours or mine would.

Aromatherapy Mistake 3: Allowing Essential Oils to Penetrate the Eyes, and Not Knowing What to Do if it Does

This is pretty obvious, but if an essential oil ends up getting into your eye, it's going to feel rather unpleasant. Avoid getting an essential oil into your eyes whenever possible. More importantly, it's important to realize that mistakes do happen. Most of us have probably gotten shampoo in our eyes while we're in the shower at least once in our lives. This too can be rather painful. When you're not prepared with knowledge on what to do when an accident does occur, then you're going to be in pain longer than necessary. You'd be surprised to find out how many aromatherapy enthusiasts do not know what to do if an essential oil comes into contact with their eyes.

The best course of action to take if you do mistakenly burn your eyes with essential oil is to avoid rinsing your eye out with water. As we've already mentioned, oil and water do not mix well. The water is going to do little to remove the oil. Instead, it will merely move the oil and swish it around in an eye that is already inflamed and red. Any type of milk is going to be much more effective at removing oil from your eye. Coconut oil is another option that you have if milk is not at your disposal when the accident occurs. Finally, any type of hand cream or lotion will also help to lessen the strong effects of an essential oil on the eye. Once you've begun the process of removing the oil from your eye by using one of the methods just described, you should then seek to flush the eye with water, removing everything from the eye as quickly as possible.

Aromatherapy Mistake 4: Using Aromatherapy Too Often

Too much of anything can become a bad thing. Aromatherapy is no exception to this tried and true saying. An essential oil is different from any other type of oil because it's far more concentrated than other types of oil are. In other words, they're stronger and more potent than oil that you use to cook with. You can certainly use aromatherapy for a few days out of the week; however, you should at the very least change use the oil in a variety of ways throughout the week. For example, instead of using the oil exclusively on your body, it would be a better idea to rub the oil onto your body one day and then use a diffuser or the steam method for the other days of the week. This way, no single part of your body will become too sensitive to the oils.

Aromatherapy Mistake 5: Being too Intimated to Start Using Aromatherapy in the First Place

This last mistake might seem obvious to some people, but you'd be surprised to find out how many people do not end up trying out aromatherapy, simply because of the fact that it seems too intimidating from the onset. There are a lot of oils to choose from, and many ways that you can go about using methods for aromatherapy. As with many other things in life, aromatherapy also requires practice and consistency if you ever hope to become truly skilled at it. Do not allow yourself to pass up on an opportunity to become acquainted with aromatherapy, even if you think that aromatherapy might not be for you. You never know until you try.

Even people who have been practicing aromatherapy for quite some time can make the same mistakes that were presented in this chapter. Without taking the time to be careful and be cautious when it comes to dealing with essential oils, injury is entirely possible. Sure, essential oils are not going to be capable of permanently injuring you, but they have still been known to inflict pain on people who choose to use them improperly. Do not let yourself fall into this same category. Be smart when it comes to using essential oils, and you'll be better off.

Chapter 10:
Getting Started with Aromatherapy

In accordance with the last mistake that was presented in the previous chapter, this chapter is going to present how you can get started in using aromatherapy as quickly as possible. The hope is that after reading this chapter, you'll have no excuse but to start bringing more aromatherapy techniques into your life. As you're going to find, getting started with using aromatherapy is incredibly easy. It just takes some patience and some know-how, that's all.

Step 1 to Using Essential Oils and Aromatherapy: Start with a Basic Oil Set

This book has gone over both beginner and more advanced essential oils that you can use in your aromatherapy methods; however, when you're first starting to use essential oils, it's best to set yourself up with only a basic set of essential oils that you'll need. Though you may think that it may be best to start with just a few oils on hand, you're going to want to be able to experiment with a few essential oils from the onset. Below is an example of a beginner aromatherapy essential oil set that would be appropriate for you to purchase:

1. Rosemary oil

2. Peppermint oil

3. Lemon Oil

4. Tea Tree Oil

5. Lavender Oil

Remember, you should be looking to purchase quality oil as soon as you decide to devote your time and energy towards aromatherapy. With these beginner oils at your disposal, you'll be able to experiment with these oils in many ways. For example, not only will you be able to figure out which aromas are your favorite; you'll also be able to determine how you best like to use oils to achieve a particular result that you're seeking with them.

Step 2 to Using Essential Oils and Aromatherapy: Get Yourself a Complementing Oil

A complementing oil is simply an oil that is going to

complement the essential oils in your aromatherapy arsenal. In other words, these are the solvents or thickening agents that we've already discussed. Without these, the result is going to be that you will cause irritation and burning to your skin. This is not necessary. Some of the best beginner complementing oils include the following:

1. Sunflower oil

2. Coconut oil

3. Apricot oil

4. Almond oil

5. Jojoba oil

With the exception of jojoba oil, you should be able to find all of these complementing oils at your grocery store.

Step 3 to Using Essential Oils and Aromatherapy: Purchase a Diffuser

This step is pretty self-explanatory. You can use the inhalation techniques that we've already discussed or the spritzing technique when you're truly first starting out with aromatherapy, but the reality is that once you become more comfortable with these methods, you'll want to have a diffuser by your side. The most powerful diffusers are those that have fans attached to them or an electric heat source of some kind.

Step 4 to Using Essential Oils and Aromatherapy: Branch Out with Your Own Recipes

Many people turn the practice of aromatherapy into a formal hobby by teaching themselves how to make essential oil blends themselves. A convenient and easy way that you can teach yourself how to do this is to purchase a book of recipes on aromatherapy (Side note, I've already written a book on essential oil recipes myself, so you do not have to look far for recipes on this topic). In addition to purchasing a handy recipe book, another option that you have is to purchase an essential oils chart. This chart is going to be able to tell you how many drops of each essential oil will need to go to a recipe to make it smell delightful. It's that simple.

Step 5 to Using Essential Oils and

Aromatherapy: Acquire Some Bottles

Lastly, if you are looking to eventually start making your own essential oils, either for personal or commercial use, it would be in your best interest to purchase a few essential oil bottles. These bottles do not have to be particularly large in size, but they should be large enough for mixing purposes. Who knows, one day you might even decide that it's time to share your creations with other people. After reading about how aromatherapy can enhance your life, it's easy to see how you can use the gifts of aromatherapy to better the lives of the people whom you love and are friends with.

This chapter has provided you with the essential tips that you will need to get started using aromatherapy immediately. As you can see, there are not too many elaborate steps to go through in this process. Even if you feel intimidated by everything that aromatherapy encompasses, stick with it. You'll soon find that the benefits that aromatherapy can offer your life far outweigh any negative predispositions you may have towards it.

Conclusion

Congratulations on making it to the end of this book, *Essential Oils & Aromatherapy: Balance Your Mind, Body, and Emotions.* At this point in the book, you should have an extremely clear understanding of what aromatherapy is and why you should be looking to use the techniques of aromatherapy in your life more often. The relaxing, yet therapeutic, abilities of aromatherapy set it apart from other types of medicine because it does not stunt the body with strange side effects or unwanted symptoms. Aromatherapy should be applauded for its transparent approach to medicinal techniques. Transparency is not something that all medicines can offer. Why not try aromatherapy techniques, rather than seeking out artificial medicines?

The next step is to take some of the advice from the last chapter and begin thinking about how you can apply it to your daily life. Remember to go at your own pace. Perhaps the best piece of advice is to see if you can do one aromatherapy technique per day for two weeks. When you're attempting to do this, the goal would ultimately be for you to become so comfortable with performing aromatherapy techniques on a daily basis that you continue to use aromatherapy techniques every day, after the trial period. Most importantly, have fun and be creative. There's no need to worry about the "right" way to do aromatherapy, as long as you end your treatment feeling rejuvenated.

Finally, if you enjoyed this book, a review on Amazon is always appreciated. Thank you again for purchasing this book!

www.ingramcontent.com/pod-product-compliance
Lightning Source LLC
Chambersburg PA
CBHW060759260726
48660CB00002B/697